WINNING THE WARDS:

ENDOCRINOLOGY FOR THE NURSE PRACTITIONER

James Lawrence III M.D.

Dedicated to our parents

Thank you so much for your unconditional love, undying support, and endless sacrifice. We love you dearly.

First and foremost, we'd like to thank you very much for purchasing this book. Our goal is to have you ultimately thanking yourself for making that decision by the time you've gone through our guide to winning the ward in endocrinology.

Because the dynamics and specific details of your endocrinology rotation will vary from those of others, it can be difficult, if not impossible, to guarantee automatic success.

Like a soldier in a war against disease, your best bet is to be as prepared as possible. At the very least, this includes securing a solid foundation of the basics of endocrinology. It also includes practicing and testing yourself.

In medicine, you can never do too much, so allow this book to be another tool or weapon in your arsenal to winning the wards!

We won't list every single thing you might need to know, but we will go over some of the most important things that help patients in endocrinology. You'll get some sample cases, some useful tables, essential tips, advice you won't find anywhere else, and more along the way.

We're always looking to improve this book to help more readers down the line as well, so if there's something we didn't mention here that you think is essential, don't hesitate to submit any pearls to us. If we end up using them, we'll give you a shout-out in future editions!

So without further ado, let's get started.

Table of Contents

Quick Pimping Endocrinology Cases: Part 1

Sometimes your attending or resident may throw you into the fire and proceed to bombard you with a series of questions.

And no matter how correct or thorough your answers are, for some reason they don't seem good enough, and the questions keep coming at you like bullet spray from a machine gun.

Don't cry. Don't fret. This surprise attack is a normal part of "pimping."

You can get ready for this rite of passage and minimize any damage to your ego by simply knowing your stuff cold.

Pretend a drill sergeant is screaming the next few pages at you (it won't be anywhere that bad in real life), and see if you already know your stuff.

Mr. Greyjoy is a 55-year-old male who complains of loss of libido, always being tired, headaches that wake him up in the middle of the night, and tunnel vision.

1. *What is most likely cause of these symptoms?*

2. *What is the best initial test?*

3. *What is the diagnostic test of choice?*

4. *What is the initial treatment of this patient?*

5. *What test is used to monitor therapy?*

6. *What is the best end treatment?*

Don't stop. No time to digest whether your answers to the previous case are right. Keep reading, student!

Mr. Snow is a 42-year-old male complaining of bilateral wrist pain, tingling of the fingers, changes in his hat size, and coarse facial features developing over the last year.

1. *What is the best initial test?*

2. *What is the next test to do if the previous one is positive?*

3. *What would you expect of the GH levels in the previous test in a normal and in an abnormal patient?*

4. *What is the diagnostic test of choice if both previous tests are positive?*

5. *What is the treatment of choice?*

You're not done yet. On to the next case!

Mr. Stark is a 41-year-old male complaining of weight gain of 40 lbs. over the last 2 months, an increased waist-to-hip ratio, central obesity, and mixed hyperlipidemia.

    1. *What is the most likely cause?*

    2. *What is the best initial test?*

    3. *What will an insulin tolerance test show?*

That wasn't too bad now, was it? Before we go through the answers, let's review some basic information as a refresher.

We'll start with the pituitary gland, which is divided into the adenohypophysis and neurohypophysis. These two parts are better known as the anterior pituitary and posterior pituitary, respectively.

Theses are the hormones that the pituitary gland is responsible for.

Anterior Pituitary	Posterior Pituitary
ACTH TSH FSH/LH Prolactin GH	ADH Oxytocin

Let's take a closer look at the anterior pituitary hormones on the next page.

Anterior Pituitary Hormone	Stimulation controlled by Hypothalamus release of:
ACTH	CRH
TSH	TRH
FSH/LH	GnRH
Prolactin	Dopamine inhibits; Decreased T4 causes increased TRH, which inhibits Dopamine
GH	GHRH

Now let's review what these anterior pituitary hormones do.

Anterior Pituitary Hormone Functions

ACTH (AdrenoCorticoTropic Hormone, aka corticotropin): Stimulates secretion of glucocorticoid steroid hormones from adrenal cortex cells. These hormones are cortisol, DHEA, and androgens.

TSH (Thyroid-Stimulating Hormone, aka thyrotropic): As its name suggests, TSH stimulates the thyroid gland to produce thyroxine (T_4) and then triiodothyronine (T_3)

FSH (Follicle-Stimulating Hormone): As its name suggests, in **F**emales FSH initiates **F**ollicular growth by specifically affecting granulosa cells, which produce progesterone. But in males, FSH induces Sertoli cells to secrete androgen-binding proteins.

LH (Luteinizing Hormone): In males, LH acts upon **Leydig** cells of the testes, which produce testosterone. In females, LH supports theca cells in the ovaries, which produce estrogen.

Prolactin: Stimulates the mammary glands to produce milk

GH (Growth Hormone, aka somatotropin): Stimulates growth, cell reproduction, and regeneration.

We might as well take a look at the couple of posterior pituitary hormones, too, on the next page. Note that the posterior pituitary hormones, ADH and oxytocin, are not produced by the posterior pituitary. They're actually made by the hypothalamus and are secreted from nerve axons into the capillary beds that supply the pituitary. Use that to impress your attending!

Posterior Pituitary Hormone Functions

ADH (Anti-Diuretic Hormone, aka arginine vasopressin or argipressin): Regulates the body's retention of water by acting to increase water reabsorption in the collecting ducts of nephrons

Oxytocin: Causes contraction and expression of milk; also causes uterine contractions during childbirth and induces labor

That wasn't bad at all. Most of those hormones already tell you what they do in their names. But what happens when hormones go wrong? Let's review some common conditions to be aware of when it comes to endocrinology.

Prolactinoma: Primary Hyperprolactinemia

1. Most common hormone-secreting pituitary tumor
2. Increased prolactin decreases secretion of GnRH, reducing FSH and LH production and causing impotence and hypogonadism in males and amenorrhea and galactorrhea in females.
3. Always test prolactin 1st
4. Sizes
   a. microadenomas < 1cm
   b. Macroadenomas > 1cm and more common in Men
   c. The larger the prolactinoma, the higher the prolactin level

Physical Examination:

1. In men, check testicles and body hair.
2. In women, look for signs of estrogen deficiency and galactorrhea. Make sure she's not just pregnant!
3. In both, check visual acuity and fields, then check cranial nerves to see whether the suspected prolactinoma has resulted in any mass effect.

Management/Treatment:

1. Give *dopamine agonists* such as bromocriptine or cabergoline.
2. *Monitor prolactin* level to see response to therapy.
3. If dopamine agonists do not yield results, *consider surgery* to remove tumor.

Secondary Hyperprolactinemia

Keep in mind that hyperprolactinemia has many secondary causes as well, including these common ones:

1. Medications
    a. Amitryptyline
    b. Phenothiazines
    c. Anti-psychotics
    d. Opioids
    e. Ca^{2+} channel blockers
    f. Metoclopramide
    g. Other Anti-dopamine drugs
2. Pregnancy – High Estrogen
3. Hypothyroidism – High TRH due to low T_3 and T_4 cause dopamine inhibition

Acromegaly

Increased GH secretion from the anterior pituitary stimulates the production of insulinlike growth factor (IGF-I) in the liver, leading to increased glucose formation and elevated blood glucose.

Patients will have doughy and oily skin, prominent facial features and folds, large hands and feet, hard and thick nails, and hypertrichosis. They may also complain about increased hat size over the last few months to a year.

Note that acromegaly is often associated with malignancies, cardiovascular problems, and respiratory disorders.

Gigantism will occur if growth plates are not fused in a child.

Diagnosis:

1. Best initial test is IGF-1, which will be increased.
2. Oral glucose tolerance test should cause decreased GH levels, but in acromegaly GH will remain elevated.
3. If both previous tests are positive, CT scan of head should be performed.

Treatment:

Medical Therapy: *Octreotide*, a long-acting somatostatin analogue

Surgical Resection: IGF-1 should be tested to make sure the anterior pituitary is still not secreting GH.

Don't forget to address any related cardiovascular and respiratory problems as well.

Hypopituitarism

Depending on the exact cause or hormone, hypopituitarism can manifest as a variety of different sets of symptoms.

First, let's see what we'd expect with an isolated deficiency of each of the hormones of the pituitary gland.

TSH deficiency: cold intolerance, constipation, and weight gain

ACTH deficiency: weight loss, fatigue, nausea, vomiting, adrenal insufficiency

ADH deficiency: polyuria, polydipsia, diabetes insipidus

GH deficiency: decreased muscle mass, increased LDL, increased heart disease risk

FSH/LH deficiency: infertility, loss of libido, (in males) erectile dysfunction

Prolactin deficiency: failure to lactate

Causes range from trauma and surgery to radiation and tumors or masses, but we'll take a closer look at more specific pathologies.

Growth Hormone Deficiency:

A tumor or mass, most commonly a pituitary adenoma, will initially cause a loss of GH. This leads to an axis-disrupting domino effect that begins with increased prolactin, then decreased FSH/LH, followed by decreased TSH, and ultimately decreased ACTH.

Consequently, your typical patient here will present with increased waist-to-hip ratio, central obesity, and hyperlipidemia.

Diagnosis:

1. Best initial test is IGF-1.
2. Insulin tolerance test with induced hypoglycemia will show low GH level.

Treatment: GH replacement

Pituitary Apoplexy:

This is hormonal dysfunction caused by acute bleeding (hemorrhage) or decreased blood supply (infarction) of the pituitary gland, usually in the presence of an adenoma.

Symptoms:

sudden and severe headache, nausea, vomiting, diplopia, ptosis, and altered mental status

Diagnosis:

CT scan should show a bleed causing compression of the pituitary gland, but MRI is more sensitive and could reveal hemorrhage not detected by CT. Be sure to check the patient's electrolytes and glucose as well.

Treatment:

high-dose corticosteroids and evaluation for possible surgical decompression once medically stable

Sheehan Syndrome:

Another type of infarction affecting the pituitary leads to Sheehan syndrome. Hemorrhagic necrosis from severe bleeding during childbirth results in postpartum women being unable to lactate. Associated symptoms, which may not appear for years after delivery, includes fatigue, lack of menstrual bleeding, hypotension, and loss of axillary and pubic hair.

Empty Sella Syndrome:

When CSF leaks into the sella turcica where the pituitary gland sits, the gland may shrink or become flattened..

Your classic case is a woman with headaches at night, but you may also see fatigue, nipple discharge, impotence, and low libido.

An MRI or CT will reveal what looks like an empty sella because the pituitary gland has been pushed to the side by the invading of the diaphragm from the subarachnoid space.

Now that we've gone over some of the more common pituitary disorders, let's go back to those quick pimping cases at the beginning of the book and see what the answers are.

Mr. Greyjoy is a 55-year-old male who complains of loss of libido, always being tired, headaches that wake him up in the middle of the night, and tunnel vision.

1. *What is most likely cause of these symptoms?* **pituitary adenoma (prolactinoma)**

2. *What is the best initial test?* **prolactin level**

3. *What is the diagnostic test of choice?* **CT or MRI**

4. *What is the initial treatment of this patient?* **dopamine agonists like bromocriptine or cabergoline**

5. *What test is used to monitor therapy?*
prolactin level

6. *What is the best end treatment?*
surgery

Mr. Snow is a 42-year-old male complaining of bilateral wrist pain, tingling of the fingers, changes in his hat size, and coarse facial features developing over the last year.

1. *What is the best initial test?* **IGF-1**

2. *What is the next test to do if the previous one is positive?* **glucose tolerance test**

3. *What would you expect of the GH levels in the previous test in a normal and in an abnormal patient?* **GH will decrease in normal patient, but GH will stay elevated in an abnormal patient like this one.**

4. *What is the diagnostic test of choice if both previous tests are positive?* **CT**

5. *What is the treatment of choice?* **octreotide**

Mr. Stark is a 41-year-old male complaining of weight gain of 40 lbs. over the last 2 months, an increased waist-to-hip ratio, central obesity, and mixed hyperlipidemia.

1. *What is the most likely cause?* **GH deficiency**

2. *What is the best initial test?* **IGF-1**

3. *What will an insulin tolerance test show?* **decreased GH level in response to induced hypoglycemia**

How'd you do? If you think you're a master already, then move on to the next topic!

Quick Pimping
Endocrinology Cases: Part 2

Of course there's going to be more of these! If you noticed that the previous set was subtitled "Part 1", then you shouldn't be surprised at all. Wanna win the war? Wanna live forever? Would you like to know more? Let's go!

Mr. Stella is a 100 kg, 52-year-old male type 2 diabetic who is currently on metformin, rosiglitazone, and glyburide, all at max dosage. His current HbA$_{1c}$ is 8.0.

1. *What is the next best thing to do to get his diabetes under control?*

2. *What dosage would you put the patient on?*

Keep your foot on the gas! Here's another:

Mr. Tucker is a 40-year-old male with a BMI of 38.2. He comes to your office complaining of drinking boatloads of water and waking up at night to urinate as well.

1. *What is the next best step to do?*

2. *What will the diagnosis show?*

3. *What are the criteria to make the diagnosis?*

4. *What is the first medication this patient should be put on if HbA_{1c} is 6.0? 7.8? 8.2? 9.8?*

Not so simple anymore, huh? Don't worry too much about that last one. We'll get to it later. Move along to the next case!

Mrs. Dunphy is a 42-year-old type 2 diabetic of 10 years who is on 40 units of NovoLog 70/30 qam and 60 units qpm. The patient reports nighttime hypoglycemia as well as fasting blood sugars of 200-300. Her last HbA$_{1c}$ was 11.5.

1. *What changes should be made to her regimen for better control?*

Yup, just one question there. That was 3 cases, so it's time to take a breather, right? WRONG. It's a bonus case!

Mr. Pritchett is a 38-year-old male with known type 1 diabetes. He presents to the emergency room complaining of shortness of breath, and his wife adds that he is not himself. His glucose is 682.

1. *What other tests should be ordered?*

2. *If K+ comes back at 2.6, what should be done?*

3. *If K+ comes back at 4.2 and ABG pH is 6.8, what should be done?*

4. *If blood glucose falls only 30 points in the first hour, what should be done?*

Now we're done, right? Never ask an attending that. Here's your punishment. It's only because we care about you though.

1. *What is the goal HbA_{1c} of a patient with DM?*

2. *What is the goal blood pressure?*

3. *What is the goal LDL if there's a history of CAD? And if there's not?*

<u>Diabetes</u>

There's a good reason why that last session of pimping was longer and harder than the first set of cases. The last few pages dealt with diabetes, an epidemic that's on the rise, especially in the United States.

About 10% of Americans have diabetes, and that percentage balloons to a whopping 25% in senior citizens. As one of the top leading causes of death in the US, diabetes costs a quarter of a trillion dollars annually. A quarter of a *trillion*, as in 12 digits separated by 3 commas! $250,000,000,000!

It goes without saying then that diabetes is an extremely important topic because you will undoubtedly come across DM case after DM case throughout most of your rotations, residency, and career.

That's why for this section we've gone beyond what you may need to know for your exams as a student. Hopefully you'll find it useful for the rest of your medical life!

What is diabetes mellitus?

Diabetes mellitus is a problem involving either the body's failure to produce enough insulin or the failure of a proper response to insulin. Because insulin plays a major role in lowering blood sugar, diabetics typically have high blood glucose levels.

Aside from gestational diabetes (when a woman with no previous history of diabetes develops hyperglycemia during her pregnancy), there are two common types to be aware of.

Type 1 DM is due to pancreatic ß-cell destruction or the inability of ß-cells to produce enough insulin.

1) Patients *require insulin* to live.
2) Patients are usually *younger*.
3) Consider screening for *autoimmune* processes because they are common.
4) Onset is not related to lifestyle.

Type 2 DM is due to decreased insulin release from pancreatic ß-cells and increased resistance by peripheral tissues to use insulin for storing glucose; this results in high blood glucose levels.

1) Patients with BMI > 25 have been found to be at increased risk.
2) Used to be referred to as adult onset, but is becoming more common in younger populations due to poor diet and…
3) Sedentary lifestyle, which along with genetics plays a bigger role in the development of DM.

Some quick notes regarding **gestational diabetes**:

1) Presents much like Type 2.
2) Occurs in up to 10% of pregnancies.
3) Both fetus and mother at increased various health risks if untreated.

<u>Signs & Symptoms in Diabetics</u>

Polyphagia: increased hunger

Polyuria: urinating excessively; water follows glucose, which acts as a diuretic in the kidneys; can lead to CKD5

Polydipsia: drinking excessively to replenish losses from polyuria

Remember the classic triad of untreated diabetes as the 3 P's!

Weakness & Fatigue: especially after meals

Weight Loss: due to the body's decreased ability to store sugars from blood in body fat

Blurred Vision: due to swelling of lens of eye; will lead to blindness if untreated

Infections: increased number and slow-healing wounds; bacteria and fungi love to eat glucose; neutrophil migration is impaired

Peripheral Neuropathy: tingling, numbness, and sometimes loss of sensation in feet

Screening for Diabetes

Patients with no risk factors should be screened **starting at age 45** and then every 3 years after that.

Criteria to Diagnose Diabetes

Any one of the following:

1) $HbA_{1c} \geq 6.5\%$

2) Two readings of fasting blood glucose ≥ 126 mg/dL

3) Symptoms of hyperglycemia and one reading of random blood glucose ≥ 200 mg/dL

4) Blood glucose ≥ 200 mg/dL measured 2 hours after a 75 gram oral glucose tolerance test

HbA_{1c} ≈ Blood Glucose Average

In a newly diagnosed diabetic, always do an HbA_{1c} because it can translate to a rough estimate of the average blood glucose of a patient for the last 3 months, as seen in the table below. Bookmark this handy page!

HbA_{1c} 7.0 ≈ blood glucose 150

HbA_{1c} 8.0 ≈ blood glucose 180

HbA_{1c} 9.0 ≈ blood glucose 215

HbA_{1c} 10.0 ≈ blood glucose 250

HbA_{1c} 11.0 ≈ blood glucose 280

HbA_{1c} 12.0 ≈ blood glucose 325

HbA_{1c} 13.0 ≈ blood glucose 350

Criteria to Diagnose Prediabetes

1) HbA_{1c} between 5.7- 6.4

2) Two readings of fasting blood glucose within the following range: 100-125 mg/dL

3) Blood glucose within the range of 140-199 mg/dL measured 2 hours after a 75 gram oral glucose tolerance test

Management of Prediabetes

1) Treat with metformin, which has been shown to decrease the progression to diabetes. Start the patient on 500 mg BID and adjust from there.

2) Lifestyle counseling

3) Check HbA_{1c} every 6 months.

Surprise Super Quick Pimping!

1. *What's the HbA$_{1c}$ goal for diabetic patients?*

2. *What's the initial metformin dose to give to a type 1 diabetic?*

3. *What do you do if a type 2 diabetic's HbA$_{1c}$ is not responding to metformin?*

1. This one should've been easy, so we didn't even bother trying to hide the answer on the next page. The goal for diabetic patients is an **HbA$_{1c}$ < 7.0**, which has been found to lower complications associated with diabetes.

2. Trick question! Type 1 diabetics are always controlled with insulin because their bodies can't make it, remember? Do NOT use metformin.

3. Medical treatment for Type 2 diabetics is covered extensively on the next pages.

Medical Treatment of DM2

When HbA_{1c} is < 9.0, a patient can be treated on metformin to get to goal of < 7.0.

1. Start on **metformin 500 mg BID**
2. Check HbA_{1c} in 3 months. If not at goal of < 7.0, increase metformin.
3. Check HbA_{1c} in another 3 months. If still not at goal of < 7.0, add a **GLP-1 receptor agonist** (exenatide, liraglutide), **DPP4 inhibitor** (sitagliptin), or **sulfonyurea** (glyburide).
4. Check HbA_{1c} in another 3 months. If still not at goal, add a third medication. This can be a GLP-1 receptor agonist or a DDP4 inhibitor.
5. If **triple oral therapy** fails, patient should have basal 24-hour insulin added to oral medications. ***
   a. If HbA_{1c} < 8.0, calculate basal dosage by using 0.1-0.2 units/kg

40

    b. If $HbA_{1c} > 8.0$, calculate basal dosage by using 0.2-0.3 units/kg

6. **Titration for insulin** is needed:

    a. If fasting blood glucose >180 mg/dL, add 4 units to basal dose.

    b. If fasting blood glucose is 140-180 mg/dL, add 2 units to basal dose.

    c. If fasting blood glucose is 110-139 mg/dL, add 1 unit to basal dose.

    d. If fasting blood glucose < 70 mg/dL, decrease basal dosage by 10-20%.

    e. If fasting blood glucose < 40 mg/dL, decrease basal dosage by 20-40%.

    f. If blood glucose is still not controlled, start prandial insulin coverage.

If HbA_{1c} is > 9.0, more aggressive management may be needed with insulin.

Caution with Metformin

As you can see from the previous pages, metformin isn't the grand panacea to DM2. It comes with some baggage sometimes, and here are a few more things to worry about when giving diabetics metformin.

Do NOT use metformin when the **GFR < 30** ml/min or when the patient has progressed to **stage 4 chronic kidney disease**. This is because the patient is more at risk for developing lactic acidosis.

STOP metformin if:

1. Serum **creatinine ≥ 150** μmol/L.
2. Patient develops **sepsis or MI**.
3. **3 days before contrast** is used. Don't resume until checking kidney function.

Common side effects: **nausea** and **diarrhea**

Other Meds for Type 2 Diabetics

1. **Sulfonylureas**: Stimulate insulin release from pancreas
   a. Glipizide
   b. Glyburide

2. **Thiazolidinediones**: Decrease insulin resistance
   a. Rosiglitazone
   b. Pioglitazone

3. **Acabrose**: Decreases gut absorption of glucose

4. **GLP-1 agonists**: Have a lower risk of causing hypoglycemia
   a. Exenatide
   b. Liraglutide

5. **DPP-4 inhibitors**: Reduce glucagon and blood glucose levels
   a. Sitagliptin
   b. Linagliptin

DM2 Medications	Side Effects
Metformin	nausea, vomiting, lactic acidosis, abdominal pain
Sulfonyureas Glyburide, Glipizide	hypoglycemia, weight gain
Acabrose	abdominal pain, diarrhea, cramps
Thiazolidinediones Rosiglitazone Pioglitazone	hepatotoxicity
GLP-1 Agonists Exenatide	weight loss
DDP-4 Inhibitors	headache,

Sitagliptin	nausea, hypersensitivity, skin reactions

<u>Insulin Sliding Scale</u>

Some patients will require insulin therapy via a sliding scale, which makes sure they have just the right amount of insulin before meals and before bed. You can impress your attending by spitting out the following steps before somebody's smartphone app does it!

1. **Total insulin units needed** = (patient weight in kg) x (0.4 if blood glucose > 200) OR (0.5 if blood glucose > 300)

    a. Example: 100 kg patient has a blood glucose of 350. Just multiply 100 by 0.5 to get 50 total units needed.

2. To get the **basal/background dose**, divide the total insulin needed in half.

Give this dose daily at night as a **long acting insulin**, like detemir (Levemir) or glargine (Lantus).

    a. Continuing the example: 50/2 = 25 units of long acting insulin

    b. CAUTION: YOU CAN NOT TAKE AWAY AND FIX LONG ACTING INSULIN! To prevent a hypoglycemic episode, consider underdosing and erring on the side of caution. Example: Trying a basal dose of 20 units first instead of the calculated 25.

3. After the basal dose, the remaining total insulin needed is given as **short acting insulin**, like aspart (NovoLog) or lispro (Humalog), 30-45 minutes before each meal (3x daily).

    a. If not underdosing the basal dose in the example so far, then 50 total – 25 basal = 25

remaining. Divide that 25 by 3
meals to get about 8 units of
short acting insulin before each
meal.

4. The insulin sliding scale isn't perfect,
   especially because every diabetic's
   body may respond differently to
   medications. That's why there's one
   final step: insulin correction based on
   blood glucose before meals. The
   higher the pre-meal blood glucose, the
   more extra units of insulin must be
   added to that meal's dose of short
   acting insulin.

Insulin Correction Before Meals	
Blood Glucose	Additional Units
150-200	2 units
201-250	4 units
251-300	6 units

301-350	8 units
351-400	10 units

What is NovoLog 70/30? 60/40? 50/50?

NovoLog 70/30 is a formulary of 70% basal insulin and 30% prandial (meal time) insulin.

For example, if a patient is on 30 units of NovoLog 70/30, then he is roughly on 20 units of long acting insulin (basal) and 10 units of prandial insulin. You can estimate this by taking 2/3 (or 67%, which is close enough to the 70% in NovoLog 70/30) of the 30 units of NovoLog 70/30 to get a basal dose of 20. The remaining 30% (or about 1/3) of the 30 units of NovoLog is 10 units of prandial insulin.

These patients normally take two NovoLog injections daily to meet their total insulin need.

If you need us to explain NovoLog 60/40 and 50/50, it's time to find another career.

NovoLog Case

Mr. Heisenberg comes to the hospital in the evening for a right knee amputation the following day. He takes 50 units of NovoLog 60/40 in the morning and 50 units of Novolog 60/40 at night. The surgeon calls you to manage the patient's diabetes because the hospital doesn't carry NovoLog 60/40, only Lantus and Humalog. He's also a lazy bastard. How would you titrate basal and prandial insulin doses to cover Mr. Heisenberg during his stay?

This patient is on a total of 100 units of daily insulin (50 + 50). He takes a total of 60 units of basal insulin daily (30 + 30). Start him on 30 units of Lantus, the available long acting insulin, to get him through the night.

That leaves 40 units (100 – 60) of prandial insulin daily (which he normally takes 20 units of each morning and night, but that's not important here). 40 divided by 3 meals is about 13 units of Humalog, the available short acting insulin, to be given before his next meal and each meal thereafter.

Yay! Math is fun when it's not an emergency and when you're not tired, right?

That case also shows you why you should be familiar with different types of insulin:

Insulin	Type	Duration of Action
glargine (Lantus)	Basal	24 Hours
detemir (Levemir)	Basal	24 Hours
lispro (Humalog)	Meal	4 Hours

aspart (NovoLog)	Meal	4 Hours
regular (IV) insulin	Anytime	4-6 Hours

Long Term Complications of Diabetes

A crippling aspect of diabetes is the wide spectrum of morbidities associated with the growing epidemic. Now that we've gone through how to treat the disease itself, let's see what can happen to untreated or highly progressed diabetics… and what to do for them as well, of course.

Heart and Blood Vessel Disease: Accelerated atherosclerosis increases the risk for MI, stroke, and DVT. In fact, **CAD** is the #1 cause of death in diabetic patients.

To prevent this, diabetics should have blood pressure controlled to a goal of 130/80 and an LDL < 100. If there's a past history of CAD, aim for an LDL < 70. Consider giving:

1. lisinopril
2. beta blockers
3. statins
4. furosemide

Microalbuminuria / Nephritic / Nephrotic Syndromes:

Testing for microalbuminuria should be ordered for every diabetic patient because protein in urine can cause chronic kidney disease and lead to Stage 5 **CKD**, in which GFR< 15.0 and dialysis is needed.

To prevent this, control HTN and give lisinopril to decrease progression to/of kidney disease.

Peripheral Neuropathy:

Feet should especially be checked at each visit for injuries, sores, and blisters.

Education on how to protect the patient's feet and proper foot attire is needed. Monofilament testing should be done once a year to check for numbness. If the patient has severe tingling and numbness in their feet, gabapentin may be given.

Eye Problems:

Diabetics are 40% more likely to suffer from glaucoma and 60% more likely to develop cataracts. Because they are at risk for retinopathy, these patients should receive eye exams at least once per year.

Infections:

People with diabetes are more susceptible to developing infections because high blood glucose levels impair neutrophil migration.

Decreased Wound Healing:

An elevated blood sugar level stiffens arteries and causes narrowing of the blood vessels. Nutrients cannot be transported to wounds for healing. The best way to prevent eye problems, infections, and decreased wound healing is by maintaining a low LDL, a BP < 130/80, and an HbA_{1c} < 7.0.

Here are a couple of things that you might observe in some diabetics. They're also some favorite pimping topics, so it doesn't hurt to be familiar with them.

Dawn Phenomenon:

This is an early morning (usually between 2 a.m. and 8 a.m.) increase in blood glucose caused by the release of hormones like GH, cortisol, glucagon, or epinephrine. They signal the liver to release glucose.

Somogyi Effect:

This is a morning rise in blood glucose (also caused by the release of hormones) due to nocturnal hypoglycemia in the night. The hypoglycemia stems from having extra insulin (for example, a patient who takes nighttime insulin but didn't eat much dinner).

Diabetic Ketoacidosis (DKA)

DKA is a medical emergency that occurs when there is no insulin and the body switches from breaking down sugar to breaking down fat and muscle for energy instead. This results in the production of toxic ketones and fatty acids, which cause a chemical imbalance in the bloodstream.

It usually evolves rapidly over a 24-hour period in Type 1 diabetics, but it can occur in Type 2 diabetics as well. DKA is also seen in undiagnosed diabetes and in patients known to have diabetes as a result of an infection, drug use, or poor compliance.

Symptoms: vomiting, dehydration, altered mental status, hyperventilation, blurry vision, fruity breath, drowsiness, cerebral edema, and even coma and death

Tests to do:

1. Blood glucose: usually 500-900
2. Urine Analysis: ketones present
3. Arterial Blood Gas: will reveal **anion gap** metabolic acidosis
4. BUN/Cr ratio: dehydration may result in an elevated ratio > 15:1
5. CBC: may suggest infection with increased WBC
6. Amylase and Lipase: nonspecific increases

The American Diabetes Association (ADA) categorizes DKA in adults into 1 of 3 stages of severity:

Mild: patient alert; blood pH mildly decreased to 7.25-7.30; serum bicarbonate decreased to 15-18 mmol/L

Moderate: pH 7.00-7.25; bicarbonate 10-15; mild drowsiness may be present

Severe: pH < 7.00; bicarbonate < 10; stupor or coma may occur

Managing DKA:

1. Start normal saline at rate of 1L/hr until blood glucose reaches 200 mg/dL, then start D5 1/2NS.
2. **Important: LOOK at potassium!**
   a. If K+ is < 3.3mEq/L, hold insulin and give 20-30 mEq of K+/hr until > 3.3mEq/L.
   b. If K+ is > 5.3mEq/L, do NOT give K+, but check it every 2-3 hours.
   c. If K+ is 3.3-5.3, give 20-30mEq in every liter of normal saline to maintain K+ between 4 and 5.

d. Administration of insulin causes K+ to shift into cells, causing hypokalemia. Re-entry arrhythmias may occur!

3. Give 0.1 U/kg insulin bolus
4. 0.1 U/kg regular insulin IV infusion
   a. If serum glucose does not fall by 50-70 mg/dL in 1st hour, double IV infusion.
   b. When serum glucose reaches 200 mg/dL, decrease IV to 0.02-0.05 U/kg.
5. Assess bicarbonate need:
   a. If pH is 6.90-7.00, give 50 mEq of sodium bicarbonate and 10 mEq of potassium chloride in 200 mL of sterile water over two hours.
   b. If pH < 6.9, give bicarbonate 100mmol over 2 hours with 20-30mEq of KCl in 400 mL of water until pH > 7.0.
6. IV insulin infusion can be tapered and a subcutaneous insulin started

when the serum glucose falls below 250 - 300 mg/dL.

7. **IV insulin infusion should be continued for 1-2 hours after initiating the subcutaneous insulin. If not, insulin levels may drop and hyperglycemia may occur once again.**

8. IV insulin infusion should be tapered and a multiple-dose SQ insulin schedule should be started when blood glucose < 200 and 2 of the following goals are met:
    1. serum anion gap < 12
    2. serum bicarbonate ≥ 15
    3. venous pH > 7.30

Patients with mild DKA can be safely treated with subcutaneous rapid-acting insulin.

1. SQ rapid-acting insulin as an initial injection of 0.3 U/kg
2. 0.1 U/kg every hour until serum glucose < 250 mg/dL

3. Decrease insulin dose by half (0.05 U/kg) and administer every hour

Hyperosmolar Hyperglycemic Nonketotic Syndrome (HHNS)

DKA	HHNS
blood glucose > 450	blood glucose > 900
anion gap metabolic acidosis	NO acidosis
ketones	NO ketones
more common in DM1	more common in DM2

HHNS is similar to *DKA* in that both have high blood sugar levels, marked dehydration, and decreased consciousness. But note the important differences in the table above.

Diagnosing HHNS:

1. Plasma glucose is extremely elevated and can reach 1,000
2. Arterial pH > 7.30
3. Serum bicarbonate > 18

Treating HHNS:

Correcting dehydration is most important!

1. Start normal saline at rate of 1L/hr until blood glucose reaches 200, then start D5 1/2NS to avoid overshooting the target glucose to hypoglycemic levels.
2. Give initial 0.1 U/kg insulin bolus.
3. Follow with 0.1 U/kg/hr regular insulin IV infusion.

4. Remember: NO need to monitor anion gap because there's NO metabolic acidosis.
5. But DO monitor potassium and magnesium, which may decrease due to hydration and the insulin.

<u>Hypoglycemia</u>

We saved one of the most common, most important, and easiest diabetes-related conditions for last. Well, let's get through this and finish up diabetes!

Hypoglycemia is characterized by abnormally low blood glucose and is due to an imbalance of insulin and glucagon release. The body may be using up glucose too quickly, or it's releasing too much insulin into the bloodstream.

As levels drop below 70 mg/dL, the pancreas compromises by decreasing insulin release so that the blood glucose may rise again.

As glucose levels decrease, glucagon levels increase to raise blood glucose by stimulating the liver to release stored glucose into the bloodstream.

The organ at most risk of hypoglycemia is the brain, making hypoglycemia more dangerous than hyperglycemia.

Signs and Symptoms:

1. Shakiness, weakness, dizziness
2. Sweating (due to elevated epinephrine)
3. Chills
4. Irritability, nervousness
5. Confusion
6. Increased heart rate and increased blood pressure (epinephrine)
7. Nausea
8. Hunger
9. Blurry vision or double vision
10. Tingling or numbness of skin

Some Causes:

1. Insulinoma

2. Drug-induced
3. Factious hypoglycemia
4. Alcohol abuse
5. Idiopathic hypoglycemia
6. Adrenal insufficiency
7. Liver failure
8. Postoperative
9. Sepsis
10. Fasting, starvation, heavy exercise

Diagnosis:

Whipple's Triad

1. Evidence of symptoms known or likely to be caused by hypoglycemia
2. Decreased blood glucose level measured while symptoms are present (symptoms usually appear when glucose reaches the 50s).
3. Normalized glucose level (> 70) relieves symptoms.

Treatment:

If patient can eat:

1. Consume 15-20 grams of glucose or simple carbohydrates.
2. Check blood glucose after 15 minutes.
3. If hypoglycemia continues, repeat and eat.
4. Once blood glucose returns to normal, eat a small snack if next planned meal or snack is more than an hour or two away.

Simple Carbohydrates:

1. Glucose tabs
2. ½ cup of juice or regular soda (not diet soda)
3. 1 tablespoon of sugar
4. 8 ounces of milk

If patient cannot eat:

1. Give ½ to 2 ampules of D50W.
2. Continue until near 100mg/dL, then switch to D10W.

3. If patient is an alcoholic, give thiamine before glucose administration.

Don't forget to investigate and treat the underlying cause of hypoglycemia as well!

It seems like it's been a long while, but let's revisit that second set of quick pimping cases on the next page.

Mr. Stella is a 100 kg, 52-year-old male type 2 diabetic who is currently on metformin, rosiglitazone, and glyburide, all at max dosage. His current HbA_{1c} is 8.0.

1. *What is the next best thing to do to get his diabetes under control?* **Start insulin for better control.**

2. *What dosage would you put the patient on?* **Start 25 units of long acting basal insulin; 8 units of short acting insulin before each meal.**

Mr. Tucker is a 40-year-old male with a BMI of 38.2. He comes to your office complaining of drinking boatloads of water and waking up at night to urinate as well.

1. *What is the next best step to do?* **HbA$_{1c}$**

2. *What will the diagnosis show?* **DM2**
3. *What are the criteria to make the diagnosis?*

   Any one of the following:

   1) **HbA$_{1c}$ ≥ 6.5%**

   2) **Two readings of fasting blood glucose ≥ 126 mg/dL**

   3) **Symptoms of hyperglycemia and one reading of random blood glucose ≥ 200 mg/dL**

4) **Blood glucose ≥ 200 mg/dL measured 2 hours after a 75 gram oral glucose tolerance test**

4. *What is the first medication this patient should be put on if HbA$_{1c}$ is 6.0? 7.8? 8.2? 9.8?*

Metformin 500mg BID; start insulin if HbA$_{1c}$ > 9.0

Mrs. Dunphy is a 42-year-old type 2 diabetic of 10 years who is on 40 units of NovoLog 70/30 qam and 60 units qpm. The patient reports nighttime hypoglycemia as well as fasting blood sugars of 200-300. Her last HbA$_{1c}$ was 11.5.

1. *What changes should be made to her regimen for better control?*

She is currently on 28 units basal insulin qam and 42 qpm. Total basal insulin is 70 units daily. Half of this, 35 units, should be her new long acting insulin dose. She is currently on 30 units of short acting insulin daily, so she should give herself a prandial dose of 10 units before each meal.

Mr. Pritchett is a 38-year-old male with known type 1 diabetes. He presents to the emergency room complaining of shortness of breath, and his wife adds that he is not himself. His glucose is 682.

1. *What other tests should be ordered?*

Blood glucose, Urine Analysis, Arterial Blood Gas, BUN/Cr ratio, CBC, amylase, and lipase

2. *If K+ comes back at 2.6, what should be done?*

Hold insulin and give 20-30 mEq of K+/hr until > 3.3mEq/L.

3. *If K+ comes back at 4.2 and ABG pH is 6.8, what should be done?*

Give 20-30mEq in every liter of normal saline to maintain K+ between 4 and 5. Since pH < 6.9, give bicarbonate 100mmol over 2 hours with 20-30mEq of KCl in 400 mL of water until pH > 7.0.

4. *If blood glucose falls only 30 points in the first hour, what should be done?*

Increase amount of insulin given in IV drip.

1. *What is the goal HbA_{1c} of a patient with DM?* **< 7.0%**

2. *What is the goal blood pressure?* **130/80**

3. *What is the goal LDL if there's a history of CAD? And if there's not?*

   Goal: LDL < 70 if history of CAD; LDL < 100 if no history of CAD

Quick Pimping Endocrinology Cases: Part 3

That's right. More. Hey, you turned the page. You felt good about the answers to those diabetes questions? Try this new set then.

Mr. Bauer is a 70-year-old male complaining of constipation and recurrent kidney stones. He has been a smoker for 50 years. Chest radiograph on admission shows a lung mass.

1. *What is the first step to do?*

2. *What is the most likely cancer?*

3. *What do you expect of the serum calcium?*

4. *What do expect of serum PTH level?*

You are called to the emergency room to see a patient who is severely fatigued, has shortened QT on EKG, and sluggish mental status. His calcium level comes back as 15.0.

1. *What is the first best thing to do?*

2. *What meds should you administer?*

Mr. Palmer is a 42-year-old male complaining of constipation and recurrent kidney stones.

1. *What is the best initial test?*

2. *If the level is high, what is the next best test?*

You are called to the emergency room to see a patient with hyperactive tendon reflexes and prolonged QT on EKG. The patient's serum calcium level is found to be 5.0 mg/dL.

1. *What is the likely problem?*

2. *What needs to be done to correct this problem?*

It should be apparent by now that the focus on the next sections is calcium. There are various causes that can be distinguished by the different changes or levels in labs. Of course it's better that you understand the changes behind each pathology, but you can memorize them if you want or at least have the next page readily available in your white coat pocket.

Hypercalcemia

Causes of Hypercalcemia	PTH	PO_4^{3-}	25 Vit D	1,25 Vit D

Primary Hyperparthy-roidism	*Incr*	<u>decr</u>	norm	norm
Chronic granulomatous disorders	<u>decr</u>	*Incr*	norm	*Incr*
PTHrP Malignancy	<u>decr</u>	<u>decr</u>	norm	nor/ *Incr*
Vitamin D Intoxication	<u>decr</u>	*Incr*	*Incr*	*Incr*
Familiar Hypocalciuric Hypercalcemia	*Incr*	<u>decr</u>	norm	norm

<u>Symptoms of Hypercalcemia:</u>

STONES, BONES, Abdominal **GROANS, THRONES,** Psychiatric **MOANS,** and more

1. **STONES:** Patients are more prone to kidney stones, nephrocalcinosis, and diabetes insipidus. Eventually this can

lead to Chronic Kidney Disease and the patient needing dialysis.

2. **BONES:** bowing of the shoulders, pathological fractures, height loss, spinal column curvature, osteoporosis
3. **Abdominal GROANS**: High levels of calcium cause nausea and vomiting, dyspepsia, pancreatitis, and…
4. **THRONES**: As in porcelain thrones. Increased levels of calcium also cause constipation and increased toilet time.
5. **Psychiatric MOANS**: High calcium levels cause memory loss, depression, dementia, apathy, and irritability.
6. **More: Shortened QT on EKG, HTN, fatigue, confusion, thirst, frequent urination, poor appetite**

Let's go over **PTH-mediated causes** of hypercalcemia first. But in order to do that, we should review:

How Does Parathyroid Hormone Work?

PTH is a hormone secreted from the chief cells of the parathyroid. PTH acts to increase the concentration of calcium in the blood via 3 primary ways:

1. **Bone**: PTH acts on Parathyroid Hormone Receptor 1 in the bone and indirectly affects osteoclasts. PTH acts directly on osteoblasts (stimulates them to increase RANKL) and inhibits osteoprotegerin by binding it to RANKL, which then binds to RANK to stimulate osteoclasts for bone reabsorption.

2. **Kidneys**: PTH increases tubular calcium reabsorption and decreases calcium extraction, which in turn increases calcium levels and 1,25 vitamin D formation.

3. **GI Tract**: The formation of 1,25 Vitamin D in the previous way acts on the GI tract to increase calcium absorption. This indirect way that PTH elevates calcium is often forgotten, and thus often tested!

Now that we know how PTH works, we can take a look at PTH-mediated causes of hypercalcemia. These causes can be further split up into primary and secondary hyperparathyroidism causes.

Primary Hyperparathyroidism:

Elevated blood calcium levels due to excessive secretion of PTH by the parathyroid gland.

1. **Parathyroid Adenoma:** 80%
2. Parathyroid Hyperplasia: 15-20%
3. Parathyroid Carcinoma: <1%

Diagnostic Approach for Primary Hyperparathyroidism:

1. Order serum calcium. Remember to calculate corrected calcium level: For every 1 point albumin is less than 4, add 0.8 to the calcium level.

2. If serum calcium is high, order PTH and look for elevation.
3. Measure urinary calcium level. Diagnosis is supported by a measurement that is greater than 250-300 mg after 24 hours.
4. Chloride/Phosphorus ratio > 33 also supports the diagnosis.
5. <u>Low serum phosphate</u> is another lab reading that supports the diagnosis.
6. Increased urinary cAMP

Remember that back on that table a few pages ago, *vitamin D levels are normal* in primary hyperparathyroidism.

Treatment for Primary Hyperparathyroidism:

Criteria for **surgical excision**, the only permanent and curative treatment:

1. Serum calcium > 1mg/dL above the upper limit of normal
2. Creatinine clearance < 60 mL/min or reduced by 30%
3. DEXA scan T-score < -2.5 at any site
4. Patient < 50 years old
5. 24-hour urinary calcium excretion > 400 mg
6. If due to adenoma: surgical removal of abnormal glands
7. If due to carcinoma: remove parathyroid gland and surrounding thyroid tissue.
8. If due to hyperplasia: removal of all four parathyroid glands, then take half of one gland and place in sternoclenoidmastoid muscle.

Surgery should be offered to all symptomatic patients.

Secondary Hyperparathyroidism:

In secondary hyperparathyroidism, the elevated level of PTH is due to a chronic abnormal stimulus.

The two most common causes are

1. Chronic renal failure
2. Vitamin D deficiency

Note: almost every patient with renal failure has hyperparathyroidism to some extent.

In addition to elevated PTH, patients will have *low to low-normal calcium* levels.

Treatment:

1. If chronic renal failure: give calcitriol and oral calcium; dietary phosphorus restriction
2. If vitamin D deficiency: 50,000-IU capsule of vitamin D-2 once a week for 8 weeks. Repeat if necessary.

Familial hypocalciuric hypercalcemia:

This is a benign hypercalcemia that is a result of a mutation that inactivates the calcium-sensing receptor in both the kidneys and parathyroid gland.

Approach to FHH:

1. Patients are typically asymptomatic, so the first thing that a clinician may notice is high serum calcium.
2. Check PTH for an elevation level, too.
3. If it's in the upper normal range, measure urinary calcium excretion.
4. If urinary calcium excretion is normal to low (< 200 mg/day) and calcium excretion rate is low (< 0.02 mml/L), give 25-hydroxyvitamin D to prevent bone demineralization.
5. Consider family history and screening.

Remember that back on that table at the beginning of the section, *vitamin D levels are normal* in FHH.

Now let's take a look at **PTH-independent causes** of hypercalcemia, starting with:

Hypercalcemia of malignancy

The most common cancers associated with hypercalcemia are breast cancer, lung cancer, and multiple myeloma.

Three Major Mechanisms

1. Tumor secreting parathyroid-hormone related protein (PTHrP)
    a. 75% of patients
    b. Most common: squamous cell carcinoma, renal cell carcinoma
    c. Labs will show an increased calcium level with a decreased PTH level
2. Tumor secreting 1,25-vitamin D
    a. Hodgkin's lymphoma and Non-Hodgkin's lymphoma
    b. Non-renal production of 1,25-dihydroxyvitamin D from 25-hydroxyvitamin D by malignant cells

     c. High calcium, low PTH, and high levels of 1,25-dihydroxyvitamin D

3. Osteolytic metastases with local release of osteoclast activating factor

     a. Breast cancer, multiple myeloma, lymphoma, Leukemia

     b. Mediated by activation of osteoclasts, not tumor cells

Vitamin D intoxication

Either 25-hydroxyvitamin D or 1,25-dihydroxyvitamin D can also cause hypercalcemia by increasing the absorption of calcium from the intestines as well as bone reabsorption. PTH is low, and phosphate is high.

Chronic granulomatous disorders

Most granulomatous disorders cause hypercalcemia. PTH will be decreased, phosphate will be increased, 25-hydroxyvitamin D will be normal, and 1,25-dihyroxyvitamin D will be increased.

The most common granulomatous causes are sarcoidosis and tuberculosis.

Treat the underlying disease when it's sarcoidosis with low steroid therapy of 10-30 mg/day of prednisone, reduction of calcium intake to < 400 mg/day, reduction of oxalate intake, and avoidance sun exposure.

Medications

Be aware that the following meds can also cause hypercalcemia

1. Thiazides
2. Lithium
3. Vitamin A
4. Theophylline

Treatment of Hypercalcemia

1. Patients with a calcium < 12 mg/dL do not require treatment, but they should be encouraged to decrease calcium intake, keep hydrated, and stop taking diuretics and other hypercalcemia-causing drugs.
2. Patients with calcium 12-14 mg/dL should be advised to stop offending drugs and to keep adequately hydrated.
3. Patients with calcium > 14 mg/dL need to be treated aggressively.
   a. Give normal saline at 200-300 mL/hour; at least 2 L per 24 hr
   b. Give furosemide to increase renal excretion of calcium
   c. Give calcitonin 4 units/kg and measure calcium to see response to therapy. Give with zoledronic acid 4 mg IV over 15 minutes.
4. If myeloma or vitamin D intoxication: give prednisone 30 mg BID

Hypocalcemia

Patients will have a total serum calcium of <
8.5 mg/dL, and symptoms will appear when
ionized calcium is < 4.6 mg/dL.

Symptoms of Hypocalcemia

1. Petechiae
2. Oral/Peri-oral numbness & tingling
3. Tetany
4. Hyperactive deep tendon reflexes
5. Trousseau sign: blood pressure cuff inflation causes the wrist and metacarpophalangeal joints to flex, the DIP and PIP joints to extend, and the fingers to adduct.
6. Chvostek sign: facial twitches elicited by tapping the zygomatic process
7. Cardiac arrhthymias: results from QT prolongation; can lead to Torsades de pointes
8. Rickets and osteomalacia
9. Grand mal seizures

Look at some of the causes of hypocalcemia.

Hypoparathyroidism: Decreased release of PTH as an idiopathic or iatrogenic consequence of neck surgery, thyroidectomy, parathyroidectomy, or radiation. Phosphate will be high, and urinary cAMP will be low.

Renal Failure: You'll see increased PTH, increased phosphorus, and decreased renal hydroxylation of 25-hydroxyvitamin D to 1,25-dihydroxyvitamin D.

Vitamin D deficiency: increased PTH with decreased 25-hydroxylation in the liver and decreased 1-hydroxylation in the kidney.

Pseudohypoparathyroidism: Because of resistance to PTH, the patient will have high levels of both PTH and phosphate.

Hypomagnesemia: Low magnesium results in low calcium levels.

Eating Disorders: Anorexia nervosa and bulimia result in decreased calcium absorption and high PTH.

Paget's disease: excessive breakdown and bone formation, followed by disorganized bone remodeling

Classic Symptoms:

1. Bone pain, joint stiffness, fracture
2. Enlarged head, headache, hearing loss
3. Bowing of legs; reduced height

Diagnosis:

1. X-ray may reveal incidental finding that first suggested Paget's
2. Serum calcium normal or high
3. Increased alkaline phosphatase
4. Normal Vitamin D levels
5. Bone can is most sensitive test

Treatment:

1. Bisphosphonates are first-line to increase bone density.
2. Calcitonin is second-line.
3. Acetaminophen or NSAIDS for pain.

Osteoporosis

Risk Factors:

1. Low dietary calcium intake
2. Immobility / sedentary lifestyle
3. Low body weight
4. Tobacco use and alcohol abuse
5. Excessive exercise
6. Increased age
7. White or Asian
8. Family history of first-degree relative with a fracture
9. Female sex
10. Long-term use of corticosteroids

Diagnosis:

1. T-score < -2.5 on DEXA scan
2. Osteopenia: T-score of -1.0 to -2.5

Treatment:

1. Biphosphonate like alendronate
2. Oral calcium carbonate 1,000-50,000 units

Other disorders with hypocalcemia

1. Epilepsy: secondary to anticonvulsant therapy
2. HIV: due to calcium chelation in foscarnet therapy
3. Chronic liver disease: defective hydroxylation of vitamin D
4. Tuberculosis: secondary to isoniazid therapy
5. Acute pancreatitis: check amylase and lipase
6. Tumor lysis syndrome: hypophosphatemia causes calcium to precipitate

Treatment of hypocalcemia:

1. If mild hypocalcemia (ionized calcium 1-1.2 mmol/L): calcium carbonate PO 1-3 g/day or IV 1-2 g over 2 hours

2. If severe (ionized calcium < 1 mmol/L) and without seizure or tetany: calcium carbonate 0.5 mg/kg/hr IV, but WARNING: do NOT give > 3-4 g IV over 4 hours

3. Hypocalcemic tetany: give 100-300 mg elemental calcium gluconate IV over 5-10 minutes, then an IV infusion at 0.5 mg/kg/hr before increasing to 2 mg/kg/hr

4. In all cases, be sure to monitor serum calcium every four hours.

Before we officially wrap up hypercalcemia and hypocalcemia, let's go over the answers to the set of cases.

Mr. Bauer is a 70-year-old male complaining of constipation and recurrent kidney stones. He has been a smoker for 50 years. Chest radiograph on admission shows a lung mass.

1. *What is the first step to do?* **Check serum calcium level.**

2. *What is the most likely cancer?* **squamous cell carcinoma**

3. *What do you expect of the serum calcium?* **Serum calcium will be elevated.**

4. *What do expect of serum PTH level?* **PTH will be low.**

You are called to the emergency room to see a patient who is severely fatigued, has shortened QT on EKG, and sluggish mental status. His calcium level comes back as 15.0.

1. *What is the first best thing to do?* **Because the calcium is > 14.0, give normal saline at 200-300 mL/hr.**

2. *What meds should you administer?* **Give furosemide to increase renal excretion of calcium. Give calcitonin 4 units/kg with zoledronic acid 4 mg IV over 15 minutes.**

Mr. Palmer is a 42-year-old male complaining of constipation and recurrent kidney stones.

1. *What is the best initial test?* **serum calcium level**

2. *If the level is high, what is the next best test?* **Check PTH level.**

You are called to the emergency room to see a patient with hyperactive tendon reflexes and prolonged QT on EKG. The patient's serum calcium level is found to be 5.0 mg/dL.

1. *What is the likely problem?* **hypocalcemic tetany**

2. *What needs to be done to correct this problem?* **Give 100-300 mg elemental calcium gluconate IV over 5-10 minutes, then an IV infusion at 0.5 mg/kg/hr before increasing to 2 mg/kg/hr.**

Congratulations! You've just finished the last of the pimping sets! From here on out, we'll still throw some cases at you, but we'll tackle them as we present them. In fact, we'll start with one as soon as you're done with all this calcium crap and turn the page.

Ms. Connor, a 30-year-old woman, presents to her PCP with complaints of excessively dry skin and hair loss. She has gained 10 pounds within the past two months despite engaging in vigorous exercise 5 times a week and monitoring her caloric intake.

What would your next step be in developing a diagnosis?

Elicit her complete history.

She reports that she noticed her hair texture change approximately 6 months ago, which is also when the weight gain began. She has gained a total of 21 pounds in the past 6 months.

ROS - positive for fatigue, dry skin, weight gain, dry skin, and hair loss

Physical Exam:
BP - 112/70
Pulse - 58 bpm
Temp - 97.6°F
RR - 12

HEENT - NC/AT, hair is dry and brittle,
PERRLA, neck supple, no thyromegaly,
Cardio - WNL
Resp - WNL
Abd - WNL

What are your differential diagnoses?

You should be thinking about the different types of hypothyroidism.

What lab tests would help confirm your suspicion?

CBC, TSH, T3/T4

That was really easy, we hope. If not, no worries. We'll make it really easy for the future by jumping into our discussion of hypothyroidism next.

<u>Hypothyroidism</u>

The hypothalamus releases TRH, which causes the release of TSH from the pituitary gland. TSH acts on the thyroid gland to cause the release of the hormones T3 and T4. The actions of the thyroid hormones are diffuse and affect almost all organ systems.

Disturbances in the amount of these hormones can lead to symptoms of either hypothyroidism or hyperthyroidism.

Hypothroidism is the clinical syndrome that occurs due to the body's response to insufficient thyroid hormone productions. Found in 2-3% of the general population, hypothyroidism is much more common in females.

The most common cause of hypothyroidism worldwide is iodine deficiency, but in North America it is Hashimoto's thyroiditis.

Primary hypothyroidism

Accounting for 90% of all hypothyroidism, the primary type is classified as the inadequate production of thyroid hormones due to an intrinsic defect in the gland itself. The causes range from iatrogenic (s/p ablative or surgical thyroidectomy), drugs, iodine deficiency, congenital, and autoimmune.

Secondary hypothyroidism

The secondary type of hypothyroidism is caused by the pituitary gland's insufficiency of TSH.

Tertiary hypothyroidism

The tertiary type of hypothyroidism is very rare and is caused by the decreased release of TRH from the hypothalamus.

When to suspect hypothyroidism?

Suspect hypothyroidism in a patient presenting with any of the following:

General - tiredness, fatigue, weight gain, delay or slowing of mental and/or physical performance, forgetfulness, cold intolerance, hoarseness, puffy face, depression, dementia

Neuro - parasthesia, delayed deep tendon reflexes, carpal tunnel syndrome, ↑ CK

CVS - bradycardia, worsening of CHF, angina, HTN, pericardial effusions, hypercholesterolemia

GI - weight gain despite poor appetite, constipation

Derm – cool and pale skin, dry skin, coarse hair, thinning of eyebrows

GU - infertility, heavy menstrual periods

What labs can be used to further investigate a differential diagnosis of hypothyroidism?

- Serum thyroid hormones: TSH, T3 (biologically active), T4
- Free T3, Free T4: you can use these if you suspect 2^0 or 3^0 hypothyroidism, or if the patient has a normal TSH despite symptoms
- Antibodies
- Thyroglobulin
- Thyroid Ultrasound
- Nuclear Uptake and Scan
- Fine needle aspiration (biopsy)

TSH is a sensitive test and is best for assessing thyroid function!

Primary hypothyroidism:
TSH > 5 U/L
T3 and T4 decreased

Secondary hypothyroidism:
TSH < 0.5 U/L or normal
T3 and T4 decreased
Variable response to TRH depending on locations of pituitary lesion

Treatment of hypothyroidism
(regardless of etiology)

Give oral T4 approximately 1.6 mcg/kg/day with a goal of TSH of 1-2. Remember to start low and go slow when titrating the dose!

Special treatment populations that may require a more conservative treatment:

Patients ≥ 50 years of age or with cardiac disease - initial dose of 50 mcg/day

Patients ≥ 50 years of age **and** a history of CAD - start with 25 mcg/day

Pregnant women and heart failure patients also need special consideration.

Hashimoto's Thyroiditis

The most common type of hypothyroidism in the US, Hashimoto's thyroiditis is the **autoimmune** destruction of the thyroid, leading to underproduction of its hormones.

Patients have **antibodies** against thyroglobulin, thyroid peroxidase, TSH receptors, and Na/I symporters.

The goiter variant presents as euthyroid with rubbery goiter before hypothyroidism becomes more evident later. The atrophic variant is hypothyroid from the start.

Common risk factors include being female, a positive family history, smoking, and high iodine intake.

Labs will reveal **TSH > 5.0** and ↓ **T4**.

Keep your eyes peeled for other autoimmune disorders in these patients.

Subclinical Hypothyroidism

This is mild hypothyroidism in the absence of the classic symptoms associated with hypothyroidism. It may be associated with atherosclerosis and MI, and a substantial proportion of these patients will develop overt hypothyroidism.

It is diagnosed based on lab results only, which will show that **TSH is normal or high** and **free T4 is normal.**

Treatment is suggested if TSH > 10 U/L.

Myxedema Coma

This is severe hypothyroidism usually in setting of other stressful events, such as trauma, MI, and sepsis. It is rare, but it is a **medical emergency** because it carries a mortality rate of 30-40%. **Decreased mental status and hypothermia are hallmarks.** Depressed function of other systems in these patients can lead to hypotension, hypoglycemia, bradycardia, hypoventilation, hyponatremia, and generalized edema.

Labs will show low or undetectable T4/T3, but **TSH may vary**. A high TSH suggests a primary thyroid problem. A normal or low TSH suggests either pituitary / central hypothyroidism or the suppression of TSH by another serious pathology or drugs like high-dose glucocorticoids or dopamine.

Treatment of myxedema coma

Give **levothyroxine** 0.2-0.4 mg IV followed by daily doses of 50-100 mcg IV and **triiodothyronine** 5-20 mcg IV followed by 2.5-10 mcg every eight hours.

Change to an equivalent dose of oral **thyroxine** once patient can tolerate oral medications. Equivalent oral dosage can be determined using this formula:

IV dosage / 0.75 = oral dosage

Only **after cortisol level** has been determined, administer stress doses of glucocorticoids (**hydrocortisone** 100mg Q8) until the possibility of coexisting adrenal insufficiency can be ruled out.

Correct hypoglycemia with IV **dextrose**. Begin empirical **antibiotics**, and monitor for and treat arrhythmias as necessary.

Other supportive measures may include mechanical ventilation, fluids and vasopressors to correct hypotension, and passive rewarming if hypothermic.

Sick Euthyroid Syndrome

This is a change in the level of circulating thyroid hormones in patients with trauma, serious illness, or stress.

It is not due to disease of the thyroid or pituitary gland. Instead, there are transient alterations in the peripheral transport and metabolism of the hormones.

Labs will initially show ↓ **free T3**, ↓ **TSH**, and ↓ **free T4** in the setting of severe illness. Repeat labs after illness recovery may show transient ↑ TSH.

Treatment of sick euthyroid syndrome

Treat the underlying disease. **Do NOT give thyroid replacement hormones** as this worsens outcomes! Thyroid function tests will normalize after patient has fully recovered.

Hypothyroidism in Pregnancy

Adherence to thyroid hormone replacement is a must during pre-conception and pregnancy.

Women with pre-existing hypothyroidism or subclinical hypothyroidism will require an **increase in T4 dosage during pregnancy**. Initial increase is usually 30% of pre-pregnancy dose as soon as pregnancy confirmed.

Some women may require thyroid hormone increase by 50% until week 20 of pregnancy.

TSH levels must be monitored rigorously every 4-6 weeks throughout pregnancy. Adjust levothyroxine dosage as needed to achieve a normal TSH.

Return to pre-pregnancy dose immediately after delivery.

Mrs. McCallister, a 35-year-old Caucasian woman, presents to the local ER with complaints that "my heart is beating too fast." She states she has experienced rapid heart rate before, but episodes have never lasted more than 1-2 minutes. The current episode has lasted more than 1 hour. She also states that she feels very hot, and she can't stop trembling.

After further questioning, you discover that she has also lost 20 pounds in the last 3 months even though she has been eating more.

Family history is positive for what she describes as "thyroid problems" in her mother.

Physical Exam:
BP - 115/75
Pulse – 110 bpm
Temperature - 98.3°F
RR - 20
Neuro: CN 1-12 intact, 5/5 muscle strength, reflexes intact bilaterally, (-) Babinski

HEENT - NC/AT, PERRLA, EOM intact, lid lag, proptosis, neck supple, no thyromegaly, no palpable thyroid nodules
Cardio - tachycardia, irregularly irregular pulse, S1/S2, no murmurs, no rubs, no gallops
Resp - LCTA bilaterally
Abd - soft, non-tender, non-distended, +BS in 4 quadrants

Based on the information from your HPI and PE, what condition does the patient most likely have?

Hyperthyroidism or Graves' disease

<u>Hyperthyroidism</u>

Hyperthyroidism is a result of an excess of circulating thyroid hormones. It can be caused by several different disorders including thyroiditis, Graves disease, toxic adenoma, and toxic multinodular disorder.

<u>Signs and symptoms of hyperthyroidism</u>

General - irritability, fine tremor, fatigue, heat intolerance, difficulty concentrating, difficulty sleeping, increased sweating, nervousness

Neuro - proximal muscle weakness

CVS – HTN, tachycardia, atrial fibrillation, palpitations. Elderly patients may only have CVS symptoms, particularly new onset atrial fibrillation.

GI - weight loss despite increased appetite, hyperdefecation, nausea, vomiting, diarrhea

GU - oligomenorrhea, amenorrhea, fertility issues

Derm - fine hair, moist and warm skin, soft nails, onycholysis, flushing

MSK - decreased bone mass

Particularly suggestive of Graves' disease are lid lag, retraction, proptosis, and decreased visual acuity.

What initial labs should be ordered?

Thyroid function tests will reveal the following:

$$\downarrow \textbf{TSH}, \uparrow \textbf{free T4}, \uparrow \textbf{free T3}$$

A **TSI** test will be positive for antibodies called **t**hyroid-**s**timulating **i**mmunoglobulins.

Also consider ordering labs for radioactive iodine uptake, glucose, and cholesterol levels.

<u>Graves' Disease</u>

Graves' disease, the most common cause of hyperthyroidism, is hyperthyroidism in the presence of diffuse goiter, ophthalmopathy, or dermopathy. More common in women, especially in the third and fourth decades of life, Graves' disease is an autoimmune disorder in which B lymphocytes produce autoantibodies to TSH receptors that overstimulate the thyroid gland.

This response can be triggered by iodine excess, postpartum state, viral illness, bacterial infections, and glucocorticoid withdrawal.

While patients with Graves' disease may exhibit many of the classic signs and symptoms seen in different types of hyperthyroidism, some that are more commonly seen in Graves' are **exophthalmos**, **pretibial myxedema**, **diffuse goiter**, a **thyroid bruit** due to increased blood flow within the gland, and behavioral and **personality changes**.

Thyroid function tests will reveal ↓ **TSH**, ↑ **free T4**, and ↑ **free T3**.

A **TSI** test will be positive for antibodies called **t**hyroid-**s**timulating **i**mmunoglobulins.

A radioactive iodine uptake test (**RAIU**) will show high uptake.

Treatment of Graves' disease

Thionamides like methimazole and propylthiouracil (**PTU**) are thyroid peroxidase inhibitors that curb production of new thyroid hormone.

Methimazole is preferred because of its once daily dosing, is more rapidly effective, and has fewer incidences of side effects. However, **methimazole is teratogenic**, so PTU is preferred during the first trimester of pregnancy, and it also prevents peripheral conversion of T4 to T3.

Beta blockers can be added for symptomatic treatment, and **high-dose prednisone** can be added in severe cases of ophthalmopathy.

Treatment should be continued until remission, which usually takes 6-18 months.

If thionamides are unsuccessful, options include **radioactive iodine ablation** and total or subtotal **thyroidectomy**. Patients who undergo either of these treatments will need to take replacement thyroid hormones for the rest of their lives.

Toxic Adenoma / Multinodular Goiter

A toxic adenoma (a single nodule) or multinodular goiter will cause classic signs and symptoms of hyperthyroidism by hypersecreting T3 and T4.

Thyroid function tests will again reveal ↓ **TSH**, ↑ **free T4**, and ↑ **free T3**.

If ultrasound reveals a nodule > 5 mm with suspicious features, then fine needle aspiration (FNA) biopsy is the next step. Any nodule > 10 mm (1 cm) will also require an **FNA biopsy** regardless of appearance.

A 24-hour **radioiodine uptake scan** will show increased uptake in the adenoma or nodules and decreased uptake in the surrounding tissues.

First-line treatment for a toxic adenoma or multinodular goiter can be subclinical or clinical thyroidectomy and methimazole or PTU to attain euthyroid state.

<u>Thyrotoxic Crisis</u>

This is an acute exacerbation of thyrotoxicosis symptoms due to uncontrolled hyperthyroidism. It can be triggered by physically stressful situations such as trauma, infection, or surgery in hyperthyroid patients.

With a mortality rate of 20-30%, thyrotoxic crisis is a **medical emergency**!

Signs and symptoms include extreme hyperthermia, tachycardia, shock, confusion, CHF, tachyarrhythmia, and altered mental status.

Thyroid function panel will reveal **undetectable TSH** and **increased T3/T4.**

CBC with differential will show **anemia** and **leukocytosis**.

Liver function tests will reveal increases in **ALT** and **AST**. **Glucose** will also be elevated.

However, **do NOT wait for labs** to confirm if thyrotoxic crisis is suspected.

Treatment of Thyrotoxic Crisis

After a baseline CBC and liver profile has been drawn, start treatment with **high-dose methimazole or PTU.**

Beta blockers will treat symptoms of β-andrenergic activity and slightly decrease peripheral conversion of T4 to T3 as well.

Radioactive iodine inhibits hormone secretion and destroys the gland slowly. If none of this works, consider surgery and supportive treatment.

Other Causes of Hyperthyroidism

Exogenous T3/T3: absence of goiter, **low serum thyroglobulin concentration**, low to undetectable RAIU

Excessive iodine: will have classic signs and symptoms of hyperthyroidism. TSH will be decreased, and T3/T4 will be increased.

Treatment: thyroid hormone dosage or discontinue. Beta blockers can be used for immediate relief of the symptoms of hyperthyroidism.

Thyroiditis

Thyroiditis is the inflammation of the thyroid gland that can cause either hypothyroidism or hyperthyroidism. It may follow an upper respiratory infection or other viral illness.

Patients undergo a classic pattern of hyperthyroidism first, then hypothyroidism, and finally a complete recovery.

The gland may be exquisitely tender to palpation, in which case you must provide immediate clinical evaluation, ultrasound, and FNA with fluid culture. Drainage and antibiotics may be warranted based on FNA fluid analysis.

Treat thyroiditis with NSAIDs, aspirin, and/or glucocorticoids.

Postpartum Thyroiditis

This is an autoimmune-induced type of thyroiditis that occurs within one year of pregnancy or spontaneous abortion.

Postpartum thyroiditis can present as transient hypothyroidism alone, transient hyperthyroidism alone, or hyperthyroidism followed by hypothyroidism and then recovery. Most women recover fully, and few will have permanent hypothyroidism.

These women can exhibit classic symptoms of either hypothyroidism or hyperthyroidism, but the symptoms usually are more vague and may even be confused with the stresses of having a newborn or breastfeeding.

Thyroid function tests will show high or normal free T3 and T4 and low TSH in the hyperthyroid phase. The hypothyroid phase will typically have low to normal T3/T4 concentrations and a high TSH.

Serum antithyroid peroxidase will be high in over 65% of women with postpartum thyroiditis.

Treatment of Pospartum Thyroiditis

Most women will not need treatment, but thyroid function tests should be performed anyway every 4-8 weeks until resolution.

For bothersome hyperthyroid symptoms, give **propanolol** 40-120 mcg/day or **atenolol** 25-50 mcg/day until serum T3 and free T4 are within normal limits.

For symptomatic hypothyroidism, start with **levothyroxine** 50-100 mcg/day regardless of TSH elevation. Duration of treatment is uncertain, but you may attempt to wean after

6-12 months and follow TSH levels to determine recovery. Do **NOT** attempt to wean if she is pregnant, attempting to conceive, or breastfeeding.

Sick of the thyroid yet? Better not be because we're not quite done with it yet, but that's one more battle completed toward winning the wards in endocrinology! Turn the page, and handle the next case!

Mr. McFly, a 55-year-old man, presents with complaints of new onset hoarseness that he says has developed during the past two months. The hoarseness coincides with the development of a nodule on the right side of his neck. He states that he noticed the nodule approximately 11 months ago, and now it has recently begun to expand. He has not had any other symptoms.

He reveals that he has a family history of thyroid cancer.

Physical exam:
BP - 120/78
Pulse - 62 bpm
Temp - 98.6°F
RR - 14
Genera l- AAOx3, NAD
HEENT - NC/AT, PERRLA, EOM intact, approximately 2x2 cm hard, non-tender, non-fluctuant mass on anterior right neck
Cardio - RRR, normal S1/S2, no murmurs
Resp - LCTA bilaterally, no wheezes or rales
Abd – Non-tender, non-distended, +BS x 4 quadrants

What are your differential diagnoses?

You should be considering the following: Benign thyroid nodule, malignant neoplasm, neoplasm of lymph node, goiter

What tests/evaluations should you order?

You should order thyroid function tests, an ultrasound of the neck, and an FNA biopsy of the mass.

The results of the tests come back as follows:
Thyroid function tests - WNL
Ultrasound - approximate 2x2 cm nodule with microcalcifications visible
FNA – Histologically papillary architecture with Orphan Annie nuclei and psammoma bodies

What is your final diagnosis?

papillary thyroid cancer

All right, let's get through these malignancies and be done with the thyroid once and for all.

<u>Thyroid Malignancies</u>

Although thyroid cancers come in many different forms, they most often present as a painless and palpable solitary nodule.

But they're not all like that, and it doesn't hurt (too much) to be familiar with some of the rare-in-real-life-but-highly-testable stuff here.

<u>Papillary Carcinoma</u>

Don't let your eyes glaze over yet though. Papillary carcinomas are the most common of all thyroid cancers, accounting for 70-75% of thyroid cancers.

Risk factors include radiation exposure and a positive family history.

They present as a hard, non-fluctuant mass with associated findings of palpable lymph nodes and **positive I-131 uptake**.

Prognosis is good: 98% survival at 10 years

Treatment for a small nodule is a lobectomy or near total thyroidectomy, while treatment for a diffuse or bilateral papillary carcinoma is total thyroidectomy.

Follicular Carcinoma

Follicular carcinomas make up about 10% of all thyroid carcinomas. They are typified by hematogenous spread and capsular and/or vascular invasion.

Prognosis is good, and treatment is partial or complete thyroidectomy.

Anaplastic Carcinoma

These are seen predominantly in elderly women who may have a history of a goiter that suddenly enlarges within weeks or months.

They will complain of pain, hoarseness, or dysphagia caused by the carcinoma's aggressive invasion into surrounding tissue.

Anaplastic carcinomas come in 3 histological variants of squamoid, spindle cell, and giant cell.

Treatment options include radiation, chemotherapy, and total thyroidectomy (for small tumors), +/- external beam radiation.

Primary Thyroid Lymphoma

These are very rare and make up < 1% of thyroid cancers. They present as a rapidly expanding mass, and patients often have a prior history of Hashimoto's thyroiditis.

Diagnosis is made via ultrasound or needle or excisional biopsy.

Prognosis is stage dependent, and treatment is based on radiation and the **CHOP** (**C**yclophosphamide, **H**ydroxydaunorubicin, **O**ncovin, **P**rednisone or Prednisolone) chemotherapy regimen.

And there you have it. Done with the thyroid!

The Adrenals

Adrenocorticotrophic hormone (**ACTH**) released from the pituitary drives the release of cortisol, aldosterone, and androgenic steroids by the adrenal cortex.

ACTH release is stimulated by the release of corticotrophin releasing hormone (**CRH**) from the hypothalamus. ACTH release is inhibited via circulating glucocorticoids released by the adrenal glands.

The adrenal medulla releases epinephrine and norephinephrine, and the adrenal cortex secretes aldosterone, cortisol, and DHEA and androgens.

Aldosterone regulates water retention, Na^+ conservation, and K^+ secretion.

Cortisol helps regulate metabolism, cardiac output, vascular tone, and Na+ retention.

DHEA and **androgens** are sex steroids primarily involved in adrenarche with feedback to the hypothalamus and pituitary.

Mr. Lannister, a 43-year-old Caucasian man who is a known Type 1 diabetic, presents to his PCP with complaints of weakness and weight loss. Symptoms began approximately 2 months ago and have become progressively worse. He has lost 6 lbs in the past 2 months without a decrease in appetite or increase in his level of physical activity. He has had no changes to his insulin regimen. He has noticed an increase in craving for salty foods. He has been under tremendous stress due to the sudden death of his mother 3 months ago. Initially, he attributed his symptoms to stress; however, he became more concerned when he noticed darkening of his skin, including the palms of his hands.

ROS: + for dizziness upon standing

Physical Exam
BP - 90/66
Pulse – 70 bpm
Temp - 98.6°C
RR - 14
General - AAO x3, NAD
HEENT - NC/AT, PERRLA, neck supple, no thyromegaly,

Cardio - Normal S1/S2, no murmurs, no rubs, no gallops

Resp - LCTA, no wheezes or rales

Abd - Non-tender, Non-distended, +BS x 4 quadrants

Derm - skin noted to be darker than on previous visit 10 weeks ago, darkening of palms also seen

Neuro - CN 1-12 grossly intact, 5/5 muscle strength, 2+ reflexes bilaterally

What are your differential diagnoses?

Your ddx may include anemia, hyperthyroidism, malignancy, and adrenal insufficiency

What diagnostic tests/procedure would you use to confirm your suspicions?

ACTH (Cosyntropin) stimulation test

Adrenal Insufficiency

✓ Insufficient cortisol and aldosterone produced to meet the body's needs

✓ Cortisol aids in hepatic gluconeogenesis by maintaining vascular tone and glycogen.

✓ Inadequate cortisol can lead to shock, hypotension, and hypoglycemia.

1. Primary: adrenal gland itself is not functioning properly

2. Secondary: ineffective ACTH stimulation by pituitary gland; can be induced by chronic use of exogenous steroids

3. Tertiary: hypothalamic dysfunction results in lack of CRH; uncommon

Mechanisms of Adrenal Insufficiency	
Autoimmune	most common; results in destruction of cortex; lymphocytic infiltration features seen histologically; Ab to adrenal cortical antigen; likely to have deficiency in other endocrine glands
Infectious	TB (most common infectious cause worldwide), CMV, Histoplasmosis, HIV (most common infectious cause in US), Paracoccidiodomycosis
Infiltrative	sarcoidosis, amyloidosis, hemochromatosis, metastatic cancer
Drug induced	ketoconazole, megestrol acetate, anticonvulsants, etomidate, rifampin, coumadin
Other	bilateral adrenal insufficiency, sepsis

Congenital	congenital adrenal hyperplasia

Presentation of Adrenal Insufficiency:

- ✓ Skin darkening, particularly at palmar crease and extensor surfaces
- ✓ Hyperkalemia
- ✓ Hyponatremia
- ✓ Metabolic acidosis
- ✓ Weakness, fatigue, weight loss, salt craving, postural dizziness, GI symptoms
- ✓ Associated with Type 1 DM, primary hypothyroidism, and neurological deficits

Adrenal Crisis

Suspect adrenal crisis in any patient with **acute unexplained shock and volume depletion**! Metabolic acidosis, hyperkalemia, hypoglycemia, and abdominal tenderness may also be present.

You must treat an adrenal crisis emergently with **IV corticosteroids**! **Do NOT delay** treatment for testing purposes!

Primary Adrenal Insufficiency

The impairment of the adrenal gland results in the loss of cortisol, aldosterone, and DHEA and androgens.

Clinical manifestations appear after 90% of the gland has been destroyed.

Adrenoleukodystrophy (ALD):
An X-linked disorder of very long chain fatty acid metabolism in which fatty acids build up in and disrupt the normal activity of the adrenal glands, nervous system, and testes

Secondary Adrenal Insufficiency

Failure of pituitary ACTH secretion can be caused by exogenous glucocorticoid therapy, megestrol acetate, head trauma induced pituitary destruction, and Sheehan syndrome (postpartum necrosis of pituitary gland)

Associated with focal neurological changes, visual deficits, diabetes insipidus, and panhypopituitarism

Addison's Disease
(Chronic Adrenal Insufficiency)

- ➤ typically has a more **insidious onset**
- ➤ General - fatigue, weight loss, anorexia, salt craving, irritability, depression
- ➤ Vascular - **hypotension**/orthostasis
- ➤ Metabolic - hypoglycemia, cachexia
- ➤ Reproductive - loss of libido
- ➤ GI - nausea, vomiting, diarrhea, abdominal pain
- ➤ Hematology - normocytic anemia, eosinophilia, lymphocytosis
- ➤ Musculoskeletal - muscle and joint pain
- ➤ Derm - thin axillary and pubic hair in females; **hyperpigmentation** due to proopiomelanocortin (POMC)

In the diagram on the next page, the pituitary tries to make more ACTH to make up for the impaired adrenal glands' lack of hormones. ACTH comes from POMC, which produces MSH as the byproduct that causes hyperpigmentation.

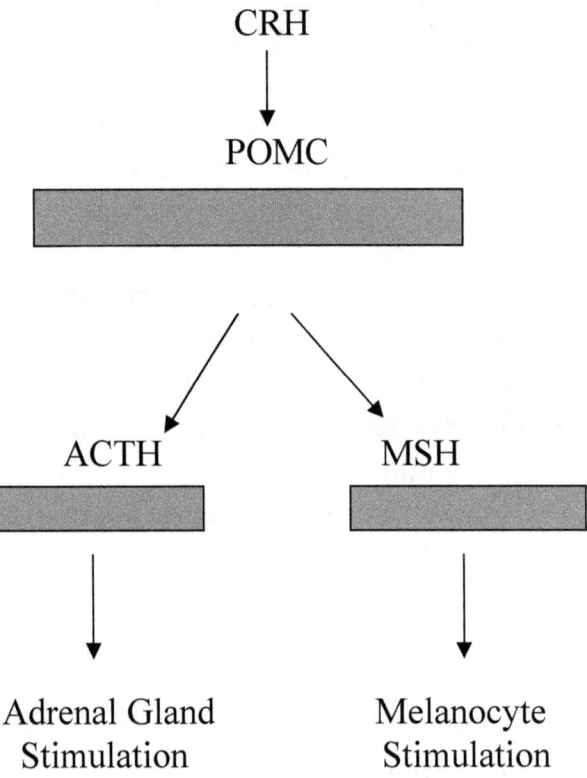

Diagnosing adrenal gland disorders can be relatively simple if the following simple questions are asked.

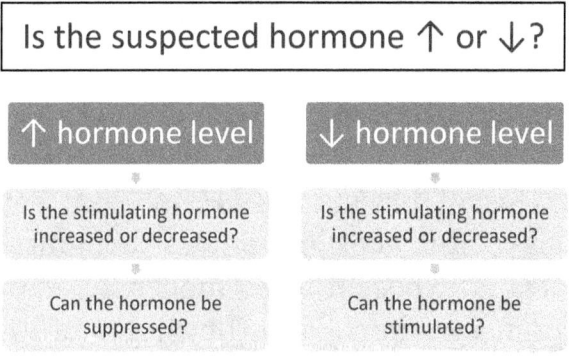

The ACTH (**Cosyntropin**) stimulation test can be used to diagnose some hormone deficiencies.

1. Measure *morning cortisol* level.
2. Administer 1 mcg cosyntropin IV.
3. Measure cortisol levels after 30 minutes and 60 minutes.

Normal response: **cortisol level > 20 mcg/dL** after cosyntropin, hence adrenal gland is responding to ACTH

Abnormal response: patient has primary or secondary adrenal insufficiency

How can you differentiate between primary and secondary adrenal insufficiency?

This can be determined by two ways.

1. Measure plasma ACTH in basal sample taken before cosyntropin is administered. ACTH is expected to be higher than normal in primary adrenal insufficiency and low in secondary adrenal insufficiency.

2. Measure serum cortisol response to prolonged ACTH stimulation. Administer a continuous infusion of ACTH (8 or 48 hrs).

   a. 8-hour ACTH stimulation test: 24-hour urinary excretion of 17-OHCS should increase 3-5x of baseline cortisol level.

b. 48-hour ACTH stimulation test: In patients with hypopituitarism (2° adrenal insufficiency), 24-hour urinary excretion of 17-OHCS should be > 9 mg after 48 hours.

Treatment of Adrenal Crisis

1. Do NOT delay treatment with IV glucocorticoids!

2. Blood draw: serum cortisol, renin, ACTH, serum chemistry

3. Fluid bolus: 1-3 L normal saline or 5% dextrose in 0.9% saline (corrects hypoglycemia) IV infusion within first 24-48 hours. Total amount infused based on volume status and urine output.

4. If patient is known to have previous diagnosis of adrenal insufficiency, then give 4 mg IV bolus dexamethasone, 100mg IV bolus hydrocortisone, or any other IV glucocorticoid can be used.

5. Seek out and treat precipitating cause of the adrenal crisis, such as infection, with empiric antibiotics.

6. Pressors (dopamine or norepinephrine) may be needed for hypotension.

Treatment of Addison's Disease or Chronic Adrenal Insufficiency

- **Hydrocortisone** 15-25 mg PO divided into 2-3 doses per day.

- **Fludrocortisone** 0.1 mg/day PO. It is a synthetic mineralocorticoid that prevents sodium loss, intravascular volume depletion, and hyperkalemia. If the patient is on hydrocortisone, then a lower dose of fludrocortisone can be used because hydrocortisone has some mineralocorticoid activity.

- **DHEA replacement** in women has been shown to provide improvement in

quality of life by having a small
beneficial effect on mood and
depression.

Mineralocorticoid Excess Syndromes

- ✓ Excess production of glucocorticoids or mineralocorticoids
- ✓ Primary: intra-adrenal cause
- ✓ Secondary: extra-adrenal cause

Primary Hyperaldosteronism

- o Excess production of aldosterone due to an intra-adrenal cause

Conn's syndrome	Adrenal adenoma produces aldosterone
Adrenocortical carcinoma	
Adrenal	Bilateral or

hyperplasia	idiopathic
Unilateral adrenal hyperplasia	
Glucocorticoid remediable aldosteronism	

Sign and symptoms

- Hypertension
- Hypokalemia with metabolic alkalosis
- Headache, muscle weakness
- Cardiovascular risks: increased left ventricle mass, cardiovascular disease

Diagnostics

1. Plasma renin activity (PRA) or Plasma renin concentration (PRC) and plasma aldosterone concentration (PAC)

   ❖ ↓PRA, ↑PRC, PAC/PRA ≥ 20, PAC ≥ 15 ng/dL
      ➤ Primary hyperaldosteronism

   ❖ ↑PRA, ↑PAC, PAC/PRA = 10

> Secondary hyperaldosteronism; investigate possible causes.

❖ ↓PRA, ↓PRC
> Exogenous mineralocorticoid source, congenital adrenal hyperplasia, Cushing's syndrome, 11-beta-HSD deficiency

2. Oral Salt loading
   a. Confirmatory test used when PAC/PRA ratio is elevated. Establishes diagnosis of primary hyperaldosteronism.
   b. Exceptions: If patient has spontaneous hypokalemia, PRA or PRC is undetectable, and PAC > 30 ng/dL. These findings alone confirm primary hyperaldosteronism.
   c. Correct HTN and hypokalemia before starting this test. Avoid spironolactone and eplerenone when using this test.
   d. Give patient a high sodium diet (5000 mg/day for 3 days) or a sodium chloride tablet can be used if dietary intolerance. On

day 3, collect a 24-hour urine and measure aldosterone, sodium, and creatinine.

e. 24-hour urine sodium should be > 200mEq to ensure adequate loading. Urine aldosterone > 12mcg/day confirms hyperaldosteronism.

Treatment of Mineralocorticoid Excess Syndromes

o Surgery is the preferred treatment for unilateral adrenal adenoma or hyperplasia.

o Medical therapy is based around **aldosterone antagonists** like spironolactone or eplerenone. Amiloride can be used in patients who are unable to tolerate both spironolactone and eplerenone.

o Spironolactone: starting dose is 12.5-25 mg daily with food. Dosage is titrated to a normal serum potassium without the use of potassium supplements.

o **Amiloride**: start at 5mg twice daily and titrate dosage to that which corrects hypokalemia.

Cushing's Syndrome

❖ Chronic endogenous or exogenous glucocorticoid excess

❖ ACTH dependent
  ➢ ACTH-secreting pituitary adenoma (Cushing's disease), ectopic ACTH-secreting tumor (pheochromocytoma, SCLC, carcinoid, medullary thyroid, pancreatic islet cell)

❖ ACTH independent
  ➢ Iatrogenic may be the most common and underreported cause because in the U.S. alone, over 10 million people use steroids each year.

> ➤ Adrenal adenomas or adrenal carcinomas (rare)
> ➤ Bilateral nodular adrenal hyperplasia

Signs and symptoms of Cushing's syndrome include round face, facial plethora, dorsal fat pad, supraclavicular fat pad, skin atrophy, purple striae on abdomen, acanthosis nigricans, HTN, proximal muscle wasting, hyperpigmentation, pathologic fractures, hyperglycemia, insomnia, weakness, bruising, oligoamenorhea or amenorrhea, hirsutism, mood disorder, and impaired cognition.

The ACTH dependent type may also have hyperandrogenism and acne.

Diagnostics

1. Measure **24-hour urinary free cortisol** to determine if cortisol is being overproduced.
   a) Normal: no Cushing's syndrome
   b) Increase > 4x normal = Cushing's
   c) Increase < 4x normal = confirmatory testing needed

2. **Dexamethasone (DXM) suppression** test as screening or confirmatory.
   a) As a screening test, give DMX and measure physiologic response to it.
   b) If plasma cortisol < 1.8 mcg/dL, then physiologic response is normal.
   c) If plasma cortisol not suppressed, then response is considered abnormal.

3. Salivary cortisol test

Treatment of Cushing's Syndrome

❖ Stop exogenous glucocorticoids if iatrogenic. Taper slowly because may have period of adrenal insufficiency when therapy stopped. Remember that prolonged use can essentially shut down the HPA axis.

❖ Surgery if unilateral adenoma.

❖ Cushing's disease: transphenoidal microadenomectomy

❖ **Mitotane** for adrenal cortical carcinoma

❖ **Metyrapine** or **ketoconazole** to treat ectopic ACTH production in paraneoplastic syndromes. These agents block the synthesis of steroid hormones.

Congenital Adrenal Hyperplasia

- Autosomal recessive
- Most common cause of ambiguous genitalia
- Majority due to 21-hydroxylase (21-OH) deficiency, which results in decreased cortisol, decreased aldosterone, and increased androgens.
- Screening for 21-OH deficiency is common at birth in the U.S.

Sign and Symptoms of CAH

- o Classic presentation: salt wasting leading to metabolic acidosis, hyperkalemia, hyponatremia, hypoglycemia, and failure to thrive.
- o Classic without salt wasting: virilizing features
- o Excess androgen production: precocious puberty, amenorrhea
- o Neonate girls: ambiguous genitalia, clitoral enlargement, urogenital sinus, partial or complete fusion of labial folds, normal internal organs
- o Neonate males: salt-losing adrenal crisis is usual presentation. Genitalia often normal in appearance but may have areas of hyperpigmentation of the scrotum or enlarged phallus.

Diagnostics

Test random blood sample for **17-hydroxyprogesterone** (the substrate for the deficient 21-hydroxylase), which should be very elevated. In neonates > 3500ng/dL is diagnostic.

Treatment of CAH

Correct fluids, electrolytes, and glucose. Give glucocorticoids and mineralocorticoids as necessary.

Hyperandrogenism

✓ Excess production of androgens (DHEA, DHEA-S, testosterone)

Etiology of Hyperandrogenism

Medications	anabolic steroids, androgens, ACTH
Ovarian	PCOS, theca cell tumors, pregnancy if aromatase deficiency
Adrenal	CAH, adenomas, carcinomas, bilateral macronodular adrenal

	hyperplasia
Pituitary	Cushing's disease, hyperprolactinemia
Other	family history, premature adrenarche

Signs and symptoms vary with sex and age at onset.
- ✓ Females-
  - o Virilization: hirsutism, clitoral enlargement, temporal balding, acne, voice deepening
  - o Defeminization: amenorrhea, infertility, decrease in breast size
- ✓ Male
  - o May have few clinical manifestations
  - o Testicular size reduction, decreased spermatogenesis

Diagnostics

- ➢ measure serum DHEA or DHEA-S in virilized female
  - o DHEA-S > 500 mcg/dL suggests adrenal tumor

      o MRI or CT to localize tumors in adrenals or ovaries

➢ If PCOS suspected, measure LH/FSH

➢ 17-hydroxylase test for CAH

Treatment

➢ Drug-induced: discontinue drugs

➢ Tumor: surgery

➢ CAH - replace glucocorticoids / mineralocorticoids

➢ Oral contraceptives

➢ Hirsutism - cosmetic hair removal.

Pheochromocytoma

➢ Catecholamine-releasing tumor of adrenal cortex, which is composed of chromaffin cells, derivatives of the sympathetic nervous system

➢ Sporadic cases more common

➢ Familial: MEN syndromes, Von Hippel-Lindau, neurofibromotosis

Signs and Symptoms

• HTN : chronic or paroxysmal

- Classic triad : **headache, tachycardia, diaphoresis**
- Anxiety, chest pain, weight loss, polyuria, polydypsia, hyperglycemia
- Any of the above symptoms may be triggered by stress, anesthesia, abdominal pressure, and tyramine-containing foods

Diagnostics

Collect 24-hour urine for catecholamines and metanephrines. Test is considered positive if any of the following is found:
  - Norepinephrine > 170 mcg/day
  - Epinephrine > 35 mcg/24 hours
  - Dopamine > 700 mcg/24 hours
  - Normetanephrine > 900 mcg/dy
  - Metanephrine > 400mcg/day

Treatment

- Surgery to remove tumor

- Combined alpha and beta blockade.
  - **Phenoxybenzamine** (alpha blocker) given 10-14 days

preoperatively. Initially administer 10 mg 1-2 times daily, then increase by 10-20 mg every 2-3 days for BP control.

o Alpha-1 blocking agents like prazosin, doxazosin, and terazosin can be used and are preferred for long-term treatment.

o Beta adrenergic blockade initiated **after** alpha blockade, typically 2-3 days preoperatively. Typically oral propanolol q6h on first day. If tolerable, administer single dose of long-acting beta blocker. Increase dose as needed to control tachycardia.

o **Never** give beta blockers before alpha blockers; otherwise you may exacerbate HTN.

- Repeat 24-hour urine fractionated catecholamine and metanephrines test 1-3 months postoperatively.

Multiple Endocrine Neoplasms

❖ Tumors of multiple endocrine glands
❖ Autosomal dominant inheritance

MEN 1 (Wermer's Syndrome)

Associated with Chromosome 11, MEN 1 affects the pituitary, parathyroid, and pancreas.

Pituitary symptoms include headaches and acromegaly if there's GH secretion and galactorrhea, low libido, amenorrhea, and erectile dysfunction if prolactin is secreted.

Endocrine tumors that may arise include insulinomas, VIPomas, glucagonomas, gastrinomas, pancreatic islet cell tumors, and carcinoid tumors.

Insulinomas will cause hypoglycemia. VIPomas will secrete vasoactive intestinal peptide and cause diarrhea. Glucagonomas will cause anemia, glossitis, rash, and anorexia. Gastrinomas cause peptic ulcers and esophagitis. Carcinoid tumors will cause flushing, diarrhea, and bronchospasm.

MEN 2 (Sipple's Syndrome)

Associated with the RET proto-oncogene on Chromosome 10, MEN 2 affects the thyroid, adrenal, and other glands. MEN 2 can be further classified as MEN 2A and MEN 2B, but they both include pheochromocytoma and medullary thyroid carcinoma (MTC).

The pheochromocytoma results in headaches, hypertension, diaphoresis, tachycardia, and palpitations.

The medullary thyroid carcinoma exhibits vague symptoms in MEN 2A but is more aggressive with earlier onset in MEN 2B.

MEN 2A additionally may involve parathyroid hyperplasia, resulting in symptoms of hypercalcemia, such as constipation, bone pain, and nephrolithiasis.

MEN 2B may also exhibit a Marfinoid body habitus (joint laxity, kyphoscoliosis or lordosis) and contain mucosal neuromas on the lips and tongue or intestinal ganglioneuromas that cause constipation and megacolon.

Diagnostics

Genetic screening - RET proto-oncogene
Pituitary adenoma - CT, MRI
MTC - Fine needle aspiration performed on thyroid nodules
Pheochromocytoma - 24-hour urine
Gastrinoma - Gastrin levels
Insulinoma - Fasting blood glucose with increased insulin and C-peptide
Parathyroid hyperplasia - Serum calcium and albumin, PTH

Treatment

MEN 1
- o Gastrinoma: proton pump inhibitors
- o Prolactin secretion: dopamine agonist
- o Carcinoid symptoms: somatostatin
- o Surgical removal of insulinoma, glucagonoma, pituitary tumors (if

medical management fails), parathyroidectomy (will not remove all of parathyroid tissue)

MEN 2
- o Surgical removal of pheochromocytoma and/or parathyroid
  - o Pheochromocytoma: appropriate preoperative medical management required (discussed on previous pages)
  - o Hypercalcemia: preoperative management with adequate hydration, calcitonin, bisphosphonates

Writing Notes & Presenting Cases

If you're currently in an endocrinology rotation, then this probably isn't one of your first clerkships, and that means you're probably already quite comfortable writing notes and presenting cases to attendings.

However, we're going to throw you some tips anyway, and they'll be more relevant to endocrinology.

It's always important to have a more concise and focused note or presentation, unless your attending prefers something that's longer and more complete. Most attendings don't have the time for that, so be efficient when typing up notes in that awfully crowded clinic or when presenting your patients during rounds.

Whether you're in clinic or on the floors, it's more than likely that you'll already have an idea of a new or returning patient's diagnosis. Just look at older notes from previous visits for hints in clinic encounters. On the floors, whoever called endocrinology for a consult should have also mentioned why.
Having this initial information will set you on the right path toward getting more relevant information for your note or case.

Once you've locked into a certain diagnosis and can rule out other differentials, focus your interviewing and physical exam on relevant positives and negatives that support the most likely diagnosis and that make others less likely.

You can bookmark the pages in this book that list the classic signs and symptoms of whatever you think you're dealing with. Of course, it's better that you know them without having to refer to those pages, and you will soon if you haven't already.

I bet that half of the endocrinology patients you'll see are diabetics, so here are some things to turn into a habit when you talk to them (some of these will apply to non-diabetics, too):

> Include information about when the patient was initially diagnosed.

> Ask diabetics everything about their medications, including the names, the doses, the times they take or inject them, and their compliance. Good patients will bring all their meds to clinic visits.

> Ask diabetics if they monitor their blood sugar at home. If so, ask them what their lowest and highest readings were in the past week. Include this range in your note or presentation later

after you report all those medications details.

Ask diabetic patients about their diet, exercise, and social history. Provide encouraging counsel if necessary.

Inquire diabetics about their last dentist, optometrist/ophthalmologist, and podiatrist visits. Do they know that they should be seeing these people regularly? If not, inform them.

See if diabetics have ever experienced a hypoglycemic episode (describe it as "feeling suddenly weak / dizzy / tired and nearly passing out"). Educate them on why this could happen (overdosing on insulin), and then educate them on what they could do to treat themselves if a hypoglycemic episode occurs (have some juice or candy). Advise them to always carry sugar tablets, which they can find in most pharmacies and convenience stores.

Don't forget to test for peripheral sensation in diabetics. That means

having them take their socks off (you
might have to help them) and touching
their little piggies.

The more you immerse yourself in the patient
encounter, the easier it'll become. Before you
know it, it'll feel so natural, and you'll have
your own system down.

By now you should be very confident in
yourself. You're a huge step closer to
winning the wards now that you've taken
care of the battle of endocrinology! Good
luck out there!